HOME WORKOUTS

For Beginners

The Ultimate Guide To Effective, Easy, And Fun At-Home Exercises For Weight Loss, Strength Building, And Improved Fitness With Minimal Equipment

ROBERT LUGO

Overview

Recognizing the Advantages of Exercise at Home:

Exercise at home has become very popular in recent years because it allows people to exercise in the comfort, privacy, and flexibility of their environment. Comprehending the advantages of working out at home is essential to inspiring people to participate in consistent physical activity and reach their fitness objectives.

The ability to work out at home is one of its main benefits. Anyone with a modest area and some basic equipment can work out at home, unlike traditional gym settings which may need travel time, membership costs, or schedule restraints. Long-term health benefits result from this accessibility, which encourages consistency and adherence to a regular exercise regimen.

Flexibility is also another important advantage of working out at home. People are free to customize their training plans based on their interests, obligations at work, or duties to their families.

This flexibility enables people to put their health and well-being first by doing away with the justification that they don't have enough time for exercise. Additionally, home exercises enable customized programs based on each person's tastes, goals, and level of fitness. HIIT workouts, yoga, cardio exercises, and strength training are just a few examples of the activities people can select based on their goals and areas of interest.

Another benefit of working out at home is that it's affordable. Although personal trainer sessions, gym subscriptions, and fitness programs can be costly, basic equipment like yoga mats, resistance bands, and weights are all that are needed for at-home workouts. Online tools, fitness applications, and educational films also provide low-cost or free advice on creating efficient at-home exercise regimens.

Fitness is now more accessible to a larger group of people thanks to its cost, including those with little money or limited travel time to fitness centers.

The main advantages of working out at home are privacy and comfort, which let people work out without worrying about being scrutinized or feeling self-conscious by others. This seclusion makes working out enjoyable, lowers anxiety, and inspires people to take on new goals or activities without fear. Moreover, home workouts remove social constraints, crowded areas, and equipment wait times that are sometimes found at gyms, allowing people to concentrate simply on their fitness objectives.

Benefits of Exercise Without Equipment:

There are several benefits to working out without gym equipment, especially for home-based fitness programs, even if gym equipment can increase workout intensity and variety.

Calisthenics, another name for bodyweight exercises, is the cornerstone of equipment-free workouts since they are so beneficial for strength, flexibility, and general fitness.

Convenience is one benefit of bodyweight exercises. Due to their small size requirements and lack of specialized equipment, they are available to everyone, regardless of money or location. Common bodyweight exercises that target various muscular groups and may be adjusted to suit varying fitness levels include burpees, planks, squats, lunges, and push-ups.

Functional fitness is an additional benefit of working out without equipment. Exercises using body weights imitate natural motions and enhance daily functional skills like bending, pushing, pulling, and lifting. By improving strength, stability, and coordination, this functional approach lowers the chance of injury and improves performance in daily activities.

One main advantage of training without equipment is its variability. Bodyweight workouts provide countless variants and progressions that let people push themselves consistently and avoid hitting fitness plateaus. Additionally, variety prevents boredom and encourages long-term devotion to a fitness regimen by keeping activities interesting.

Exercise without the use of equipment increases proprioception and body awareness. People doing bodyweight exercises need to focus on appropriate form and alignment, maintain balance, and activate their stabilizer muscles. This increased awareness enhances general body control and neuromuscular coordination by improving posture, movement efficiency, and kinesthetic sensibility.

Exercises without equipment also have the benefit of being versatile.

You can work out with bodyweight exercises anywhere, whether it's at home, outside, on the road, or in confined locations. This adaptability makes it impossible to cite a lack of equipment or gym access as an excuse for skipping workouts, enabling people to maintain consistency in their fitness routines.

Goal-Setting for Exercises at Home:

Establishing attainable goals is crucial to getting the most out of at-home workouts and maintaining motivation as you progress toward your fitness objectives. Establishing goals gives people focus, direction, and a sense of purpose as they lead them toward measurable results and advancement.

It's crucial to use the SMART criteria—Specific, Measurable, Achievable, Relevant, and Time-bound—while establishing goals for at-home workouts.

Certain objectives, such as reaching a weight loss target, building muscle mass, enhancing cardiovascular fitness, or becoming an expert at a certain exercise, specify precisely what you want to accomplish. Measurable goals include measurable criteria, like lifting greater weight, doing more reps, or cutting down on workout time that let you monitor your progress objectively.

Achievable goals take into account your existing fitness level, time constraints, and available resources to ensure that they are both reasonable and achievable. Achievable goals foster confidence and drive towards more ambitious goals, whereas unrealistic goals might cause frustration or burnout.

Relevant objectives complement your beliefs, lifestyle, and overall fitness goals. They ought to have purpose and support your long-term health, happiness, and development on a personal level. Time-bound objectives have a set deadline, which fosters accountability and a sense of urgency.

This period can be used to accomplish short-term objectives like finishing a certain exercise regimen in six weeks or long-term objectives like reaching a particular level of fitness in a year.

Establishing a Helpful Environment

Home workouts are much more successful when they take place in a supportive setting that offers encouragement, accountability, and positive reinforcement. Establishing a helpful workplace requires the following crucial tactics:

1. Establishing a Specific Area for Exercise: Setting aside space for exercise helps to mentally and physically divide exercise time from other pursuits.

This area needs to be well-ventilated, distraction-free, and furnished with all the equipment you need for your workouts.

2. Recruiting Social Support: By disclosing your fitness objectives to loved ones, coworkers, or friends, you can build a network of support that promotes accountability, inspiration, and friendship.

Participating in online groups, group classes, or virtual fitness challenges can also help to create a supportive and connected environment.

3. Creating a Routine: Reaching your fitness objectives requires consistency. Whether you work out every day, a few times a week, or on particular days, developing a regular exercise schedule will help you develop discipline, habits, and forward momentum. It's also simpler to prioritize exercise over other obligations when you set regular training times.

4. Celebrating Milestones: Acknowledging and honoring successes, advancements, and milestones on the path to fitness encourages healthy habits and increases drive. This can be giving yourself a treat when you meet a particular objective, praising yourself for gains in stamina or strength, or celebrating victories with those in your support system.

5. Seeking Professional counsel: Fitness experts, such as personal trainers, dietitians, or physical

therapists, can offer specialized counsel, individualized workout regimens, and expert supervision. A professional's attention to each person's needs and objectives improves the safety, efficacy, and enjoyment of at-home exercises.

CHAPTER 1
Principles Of Home Workouts

Exercise routines at home are designed with a few fundamental ideas in mind to maximize both safety and efficacy. Specificity is a key concept that allows exercises to be customized to each person's fitness level. This theory emphasizes focusing on particular muscle groups or motions that are associated with desired results, such as increasing flexibility, strength, or endurance. Focusing on particular areas can make at-home workouts more effective and goal-oriented.

Progressive overload, which is progressively raising the volume, length, or intensity of workouts to continuously test the body, is another important concept. This idea prevents plateaus and promotes cardiovascular endurance or muscle growth to guarantee continuous adaptation and improvement. Progressive overload can be accomplished by varying the resistance, increasing the number of repetitions or sets, or introducing more difficult workout variations.

When it comes to at-home workouts, consistency is essential since it highlights the value of regularity and commitment to a fitness regimen. Long-term fitness improvements are facilitated by consistency because it enable the body to adjust to training stimuli and respond favorably. Beyond just increasing physical fitness, it also develops healthy habits and discipline, which add to general well-being.

Comprehending the Fundamentals of Progressive Overload: A fundamental idea in fitness training, which encompasses at-home exercises, is progressive overload. It centers on the notion of progressively raising the demands made on the body to promote improvement and adaptation.

To achieve constant improvement and prevent performance plateaus, this principle is crucial.

Increasing resistance is a component of progressive overload and can be accomplished in several ways, including by adding weights, utilizing resistance bands, or changing one's body position to make the exercise more challenging. Progressive overload helps muscles grow, builds strength, and improves function by pushing them beyond their present capabilities.

The control of intensity and volume is another aspect of progressive overload. You can improve your endurance and performance by gradually overloading your muscles and cardiovascular system with more repetitions, sets, or frequency of workouts. Similarly, varying the intensity by adding high-intensity intervals or more difficult workout variations can push the body to new limits and encourage additional adaptations from the body.

Importance of Variation and Adaptation: To encourage ongoing improvement and avoid stagnation, home workouts must incorporate these two essential concepts. Exercise regimens that are varied not only maintain their interest and engagement but also guarantee thorough muscle stimulation and skill improvement.

Changes in workout formats, equipment experiments, and training modalities are just a few examples of how variation can be incorporated into a routine. People can target different muscle areas, lower their risk of overuse problems, and keep their enthusiasm levels high by constantly varying up their workouts and forms.

The body responds to training stimuli through adaptation, which results in physiological changes that raise fitness levels. Exercises at home should be planned to help with adaptation by gradually pushing the body, giving enough time for rest, and including healthy food and fluids.

A better understanding of the body's response to various stimuli enables the design of workouts and the optimization of training results.

Cardiovascular and Strength Training Balance: For complete fitness growth during at-home workouts, striking a balance between cardiovascular and strength training is crucial. Cardiovascular workouts increase heart health, endurance, and calorie expenditure. Examples of these exercises include jogging, cycling, and jump rope. However, strength training activities increase muscle strength, power, and functional ability. These exercises include bodyweight exercises, resistance training, and weightlifting.

Combining the two forms of training into a workout program while accounting for personal preferences, fitness levels, and goals constitutes a balanced approach. To achieve balance and maximize workout efficiency, try circuit training, interval training, or hybrid workouts that incorporate strength and aerobic routines. Additionally, by enhancing the range of motion, joint health, and movement quality, adding flexibility and mobility exercises to the regimen improves overall fitness.

Including Flexibility and Mobility: These two aspects are vital to at-home exercise regimens that enhance general health and fitness but are frequently disregarded. While mobility includes both joint functionality and movement quality, flexibility refers to the ability of muscles and joints to move through their entire range of motion.

Stretching, yoga, and Pilates are examples of flexibility exercises that help increase muscle elasticity, decrease muscle tension, and reduce the risk of injury. Major muscle group stretches can improve posture, flexibility, and joint health, which can improve overall movement mechanics and athletic performance.

The goals of mobility exercises are to improve motor control, stability, and joint mobility. Dynamic movements, mobility drills, and corrective exercises that target certain movement patterns or imbalances are frequently included in these workouts.

People can enhance their functional movement, lower their risk of injury, and maximize their physical performance in a variety of activities by adding mobility work into their at-home workout regimens.

CHAPTER 2
Exercises for body weight

The foundation of at-home workouts is bodyweight exercises, which provide an adaptable and affordable means of enhancing strength, endurance, and general fitness without the need for specialized gear. These exercises are appropriate for people of all fitness levels and abilities because they use the body's weight as resistance. Individuals can build full-body and specific muscle group workouts, explore basic bodyweight exercises, comprehend progressions and adaptations, and develop effective and varied home training routines to meet their fitness goals.

Any at-home training regimen starts with basic bodyweight movements. These exercises, which work for several muscular groups at once, usually consist of motions like planks, push-ups, squats, and lunges. For example, squats work the quadriceps, hamstrings, glutes, and core, which makes them a great exercise for building strength in the lower body and functional movement patterns. Conversely, lunges improve leg strength, balance, and coordination, which helps with lower body mobility and stability. Planks work the core muscles, which include the lower back, oblique's, and abdominals. Push-ups are a traditional upper body workout that works the chest, shoulders, and triceps. By learning these essential bodyweight exercises, individuals can create a solid platform for more complex routines and progressions.

Progressions and adaptations play a significant role in customizing bodyweight exercises to suit different fitness levels and goals. Progressions involve increasing the difficulty or intensity of activity to continue pushing the muscles and fostering growth. For example, moving up to jump squats from conventional squats adds a plyometric component that increases explosiveness and power. Likewise, increasing the difficulty of normal push-ups to one-arm or diamond push-ups puts more strain on the triceps and chest muscles.

Conversely, modifications enable people to modify activities to account for limits, injuries, or differences in strength. For instance, people with wrist problems or those just starting can benefit from doing wall push-ups or knee push-ups to strengthen their upper bodies. Comprehending the appropriate integration of advancements and adjustments guarantees a comprehensive and versatile at-home exercise regimen.

Full-body bodyweight exercises are extensive regimens that work for several muscle groups in one session, making them a quick and efficient technique to increase general fitness.

These exercises usually consist of a mix of compound movements that engage multiple body parts at once. For instance, burpees, mountain climbers, jumping jacks, and plank variations can all be included in a full-body bodyweight workout to create a dynamic and difficult regimen that improves strength, endurance, and cardiovascular fitness.

Exercises targeting the upper body, lower body, and core can help people attain a well-rounded, holistic workout that targets different aspects of fitness.

Targeted muscle group exercises concentrate on particular body parts, enabling people to prioritize muscular growth, enhance strength, and meet particular fitness objectives. Exercises like push-ups, pull-ups, dips, and arm variations like bodyweight resistance tricep dips or bicep curls are frequently included in upper-body training.

To target the quadriceps, hamstrings, glutes, and calves, lower body exercises may include squats, lunges, calf lifts, and leg raises. To build strength in the abdominals, obliques, and lower back muscles, core-focused exercises include planks, Russian twists, bicycle crunches, and leg lifts. People can successfully address areas of strength or weakness and achieve balanced muscular development by customizing their workouts to target specific muscle groups.

 bodyweight exercises provide a flexible and efficient method for at-home workouts that enables people to increase their strength, stamina, and general fitness without the need for any equipment. Through comprehension of basic bodyweight exercises, the integration of progressions and adaptations, and the creation of full-body and targeted muscle group workouts, people can craft comprehensive and customized home workout regimens that suit their fitness objectives and inclinations. Bodyweight exercises are an essential part of any at-home fitness program because they can significantly increase physical fitness with regular practice and growth.

CHAPTER 3
Workouts For The Heart And Lungs

Exercises involving the heart are essential to every fitness program, including those done at home. The purpose of these exercises is to increase heart rate, enhance cardiovascular endurance, and support heart health in general.

High-Intensity Interval Training is one of the best at-home cardiovascular exercise techniques (HIIT). Short bursts of intensive activity are interspersed with rest or low-intensity exercise during high-intensity interval training (HIIT). This kind of exercise is a good option for people who are short on time because it increases metabolic rate and calorie burn in addition to improving cardiovascular fitness.

You can use HIIT in a variety of ways in your at-home exercise program. For instance, you can quickly switch between exercises like burpees, jumping jacks, high knees, and mountain climbers, and then take short breaks or actively recover by walking or running slowly in place. This method provides a thorough workout in less time by taxing your cardiovascular system and working a variety of muscle groups.

Many low-impact aerobic workouts are available that may be performed at home without causing undue strain on the joints for those seeking low-impact alternatives. Walking, cycling, swimming (if you have access to a pool), and using cardio equipment like ellipticals or rowing machines are examples of low-impact aerobic exercises.

These exercises are ideal for people with joint problems or those recuperating from accidents since they are easier on the joints while yet having significant cardiovascular benefits.

Another effective technique to add cardiovascular training to your at-home fitness regimen is Tabata workouts. The exact regimen for Tabata training consists of eight rounds, or twenty seconds of intense exercise followed by ten seconds of recovery.

With this approach, you can work hard throughout the work intervals and take short breaks for recovery. Exercises like lunges, push-ups, sprints, and squats can be used to design a Tabatha session that works your cardiovascular system and strength simultaneously.

Another efficient technique for improving cardiovascular health and complete body conditioning at home is circuit training. Circuit training is doing a set of exercises back-to-back with little to no break in between. This works for several muscle groups and raises your heart rate throughout the exercise, which improves your strength and cardiovascular health. Strength activities like planks, push-ups, and squats can be combined with aerobic workouts like jumping rope, high knees, and mountain climbers to create a circuit.

This combo guarantees a complete workout that improves muscle strength and endurance.

there are several ways to include cardiovascular activities in your at-home workout program, including Tabatha workouts, circuit training, high-intensity interval training, and low-impact cardio exercises. These choices accommodate varying fitness levels and objectives by allowing for flexibility in workout intensity. You may strengthen your heart, increase your endurance, and improve your general fitness from the comfort of your own home by selecting the ideal combination of cardiovascular workouts and adding them to your routine regularly.

CHAPTER 4
Adaptability And Mobility

Increased mobility and flexibility are essential for improving the efficiency and security of at-home exercise programs. Gaining an understanding of these ideas can have a big influence on your fitness path. While mobility includes both the range of motion and the control and stability within it, flexibility refers to the ability of muscles and joints to move over their whole range of motion. When it comes to at-home training, an emphasis on mobility and flexibility can result in increased performance, a lower chance of injury, and better overall movement quality.

There are various important things to consider when it comes to the significance of flexibility and mobility in at-home workouts. First of all, adding flexibility exercises to your routine can help preserve and enhance the health of your joints by alleviating stiffness and producing more synovial fluid, which lubricates them.

This is particularly crucial for people who lead sedentary lifestyles or spend a lot of time sitting down since it mitigates the damaging effects of prolonged sitting on posture and mobility.

Exercises for mobility and flexibility also help to improve muscular balance and coordination, both of which are necessary for appropriate movement patterns during workouts. Additionally, they support improved muscle recruitment and activation, which results in strength training sessions that are more successful. For instance, improved hip mobility can lead to better squat form and depth, which in turn improves glute and quadriceps engagement.

One of the most important things you can do to increase your flexibility at home is to incorporate stretching exercises. Over time, static stretching—which involves holding a muscle extended for a certain amount of time—helps to lengthen muscles and increase flexibility.

In contrast, dynamic stretching is a useful technique for increasing mobility and warming up before activity because it allows muscles and joints to go through their whole range of motion under controlled circumstances.

Furthermore, by emphasizing motions that test stability and range of motion, mobility drills particularly target joint health and functionality. These exercises can be customized to target particular body parts and frequently imitate real-life actions. Exercises like overhead presses and pull-ups benefit from an improved overhead range of motion, which can be achieved with shoulder mobility drills.

Self-myofascial release methods and foam rolling are useful tools for improving range of motion and flexibility at home. By applying pressure to tense or aching muscles using a foam roller, you can relieve tension and enhance blood flow to the affected area.

This can be especially helpful in relieving muscle stiffness from prolonged sitting or following vigorous exercise.

Furthermore, including dynamic mobility tasks in your warm-up will help your body get ready for exercise and reduce the risk of injury. To engage muscles and increase joint mobility, these drills require going across a variety of planes of action, such as lunges with rotations or leg swings.

mobility and flexibility are critical elements of successful at-home exercise regimens. Through comprehension of their significance and integration of mobility exercises, self-myofascial release methods, and stretching procedures, you can strengthen muscle coordination, improve joint health, and maximize your overall fitness performance.

CHAPTER 5
Progress Monitoring And Objective Establishment

Setting goals and monitoring your progress are essential components of a productive at-home exercise program. Tracking progress enables modifications and maintains motivation levels while setting specific, quantifiable goals gives direction and drive. Setting quantifiable objectives for at-home workouts requires careful consideration of several crucial elements.

First and foremost, objectives ought to be clear and doable. Specific targets, like "increase muscle mass by 5% in three months" or "run a 5k in under 30 minutes," are more beneficial than general ones like "get fit." Specific goals give you a clear focus and make it easier to monitor your progress.

Second, objectives ought to be quantifiable. This implies that to track progress impartially, they should be quantifiable. Measurable data can be obtained to evaluate progress, for instance, by documenting exercise performance with apps or journals or by measuring changes in body composition with instruments like body fat calipers.

Objectives should also be reachable in a reasonable amount of time. Impossible ambitions can cause demotivation and frustration. It's critical to take into account elements like your present level of fitness, the time you have available for exercise, and any obstacles or constraints that can hinder your progress.

After objectives are set, monitoring advancement becomes essential. This can be achieved in several ways, including by planning routine evaluations like fitness tests or body measures, utilizing fitness tracking applications, or keeping an exercise log. Monitoring development makes it possible to continuously assess performance and pinpoint areas that might require improvement.

The secret to continuous improvement is modifying the exercise regimen in light of progress monitoring. If objectives are being reached too quickly, it might be necessary to step up the effort or take on more difficult tasks. On the other side, changes like modifying workout frequency, intensity, or activity selection can be required if progress isn't happening as quickly as anticipated.

It's critical to recognize and celebrate your progress to keep yourself motivated and dedicated to your at-home exercise regimen. Whether it's hitting a weight reduction goal, beating a personal record during a workout, or learning a new exercise, recognizing and celebrating successes raises spirits and strengthens the sense of achievement.

It can be difficult to maintain motivation while working out at home, but recognizing accomplishments, making new objectives, and monitoring your progress are useful tactics.

People can stay motivated and succeed long-term with at-home exercise regimens by setting measurable goals, monitoring their progress, making necessary adjustments, and applauding their accomplishments.

CHAPTER 6
Diet And At-Home Exercises

To complement the effectiveness of at-home workouts, nutrition is essential.

The energy and nutrients required for physical exercise, muscle regeneration, and general well-being are obtained from the food we eat. Understanding the significance of nutrition becomes even more important when it comes to at-home workouts because it has a direct impact on exercise performance, recovery, and long-term progress.

Nutritional practices before exercise are crucial for maximizing results from at-home workouts.

A well-balanced breakfast or snack that includes healthy fats, carbohydrates, and protein in moderation can supply the energy and nutrition needed to power an exercise routine. Since carbohydrates are the main fuel supply for intense exercise, they are especially significant.

Maintaining energy levels during the exercise session can be achieved by including complex carbs in the pre-workout meal, such as whole grains, fruits, and vegetables.

Consuming protein before working out at home is essential for maintaining and repairing muscle. Eating a snack or meal high in protein can assist avoid the breakdown of muscles during exercise and encourage the growth and healing of muscles afterward.

Lean meats, chicken, fish, eggs, dairy products, legumes, and plant-based protein sources like tofu and tempeh are all excellent sources of protein before working out.

Hydration is just as important to pre-workout nutrition as macronutrients. Since dehydration can cause fatigue, decreased endurance, and cognitive impairment, maintaining proper hydration is essential for peak performance. Before working out, consuming a sufficient amount of water promotes temperature regulation, fluid balance, and increased exercise capacity.

Nutrition after exercise is also crucial to optimizing the advantages of at-home training. The body needs nutrition to restore glycogen stores, heal injured muscles, and aid in recovery after an exercise.

It is advised to have a combination of protein and carbohydrates during the post-workout window, which is usually between 30 and 60 minutes after exercise, to promote muscle growth and recuperation.

Protein offers the amino acids required for muscle synthesis and repair, while carbohydrates aid in the replenishment of glycogen stores.

Incorporating carbohydrates that digest quickly, like fruits, rice cakes, or sports drinks, helps hasten the process of replenishing glycogen.

You can improve muscle protein synthesis and recovery by combining carbs with a high-quality protein source, such as Greek yogurt, whey protein, or a protein smoothie.

After an exercise, staying hydrated is still crucial to replenishing fluids lost through perspiration and promoting the healing process.

It may also be necessary to restore electrolytes like salt, potassium, and magnesium, particularly after strenuous or extended activity sessions. Maintaining electrolyte balance and promoting recovery can be achieved by consuming electrolyte-rich fluids or by mixing electrolyte supplements into post-workout drinks.

Improving nutrition before and after at-home workouts is crucial for reaching fitness objectives, boosting performance, and promoting muscle recovery.

Meals before exercise should have a good ratio of protein and carbs to fuel the body and assist the muscles. Meals after exercise should refill glycogen stores, encourage muscle regeneration, and hydrate the body for maximum recovery.

The efficacy of at-home exercise regimens can be further increased by customizing dietary plans to meet specific needs and levels of exercise intensity.

CHAPTER 7
Overcoming Obstacles

Compared to working out at the gym or outside, working out at home poses different problems.

The absence of specialized equipment and space limitations are two significant obstacles. Without easy access to a large selection of weights or equipment, people can find it difficult to efficiently target particular muscle areas. Additionally, interruptions from domestic duties or family obligations can lessen the constancy of exercise routines. Furthermore, in the absence of a social support system or an external gym setting, motivation may decline.

typical problems with Home Workouts: Home fitness regimens may be hampered by several typical problems. One common problem is that exercises aren't varied enough, which eventually causes boredom and lower interest. Another issue is the tendency to put off or forego workouts since one views home more as a place to unwind than as a place to work out. Inadequate understanding of correct form and technique can also restrict the effectiveness of workouts and raise the risk of injury. Lastly, finding time for a regular workout might be difficult while juggling caregiving obligations or work-from-home schedules.

Methods for Maintaining Discipline and Consistency: For at-home workouts to be effective, discipline and consistency are essential. Establishing a set exercise regimen and treating it as a non-negotiable professional commitment is one useful tactic.

Having well-defined and quantifiable objectives can also boost motivation and give a feeling of achievement. Further reinforcing consistency is the use of fitness tracking apps or online forums for accountability. Additionally, you may avoid boredom and sustain interest over time by adding diversity to your workouts by experimenting with different activities or workout forms.

Benefits of Regular Exercise for Mental Health: Regular exercise, especially at-home workouts, has a positive impact on mental health. Endorphins are neurotransmitters that are produced in response to physical activity and are linked to emotions of happiness and well-being. By encouraging relaxation and reducing cortisol levels, exercise also lessens stress.

In addition, regular exercise can strengthen cognitive function, increase self-esteem, and improve the quality of sleep. Getting moving at home is an easy and accessible method to benefit from these mental health advantages.

Establishing a Supportive Workout Atmosphere at Home: A good exercise regimen depends on having a supportive atmosphere at home. Even if it's just a tiny corner of a room, designating a specific area for exercise might help you mentally mark the beginning of a workout.

Eliminating distractions from the gym, such as electrical gadgets and noisy surroundings, helps enhance attention and concentration. Motivating components like motivational phrases or images can help improve motivation and attitude. Last but not least, working out with relatives or roommates can promote a sense of support and togetherness.

CHAPTER 8
Special Remarkable

Special Considerations for Home Workouts: It's important to take into account several aspects when creating home workout programs because these can affect the safety and efficacy of the exercises.

Special considerations cover a wide range of topics, such as participant age, how to fit workouts into hectic schedules, how to modify exercises for small spaces, and how to prevent and recover from injuries. Every one of these factors is essential in guaranteeing that at-home exercises are not just doable but also advantageous in enhancing physical health and overall well-being.

Home Workouts for Various Age Groups: It's Critical to Customise Home Workouts for Various Age Groups to Optimise Benefits and Reduce Injury Risk. For kids, the focus should be on enjoyable and captivating activities that encourage the growth of motor skills and general physical exercise. A combination of cardiovascular, strength, and flexibility exercises tailored to an adult's fitness level and goals might be beneficial. Exercises that target balance, mobility, and joint health are essential for seniors. Safety and progressive progression are key components in preventing falls and injuries.

Fitting Home Exercises into Busy Schedules: Finding the time to work out amid busy schedules is a common problem people have while attempting at-home exercises. Time management strategies, such as arranging exercises during less busy times, dividing sessions into shorter intervals throughout the day, and emphasizing physical activity as a non-negotiable component of daily routine, are strategies for implementing home workouts. Additionally, you can maximize results in a short amount of time by choosing effective and efficient workout programs that target several muscle groups.

Creating Workout Plans with Limited Area: Having a tiny area is a major barrier to at-home exercise, particularly in cities or smaller homes. Workout modifications for small spaces require imagination and ingenuity. It can be useful to use bodyweight workouts like push-ups, squats, and planks that require little equipment. Multipurpose equipment, such as adjustable dumbbells or resistance bands, provides for a range of exercises without requiring a lot of room. Exercises that involve jumping rope or using the wall to exercise maximize the use of available space.

Handling Injury Prevention and Recovery: To guarantee long-term adherence and success, injury prevention must be given top priority in at-home workouts. This entails following appropriate warm-up and cool-down schedules, increasing volume and intensity gradually, performing exercises with correct form and technique, and paying attention to your body's cues to prevent overtraining.

For a safe and long-lasting fitness journey, it is crucial to apply suitable recovery measures, such as rest, ice, compression, and elevation (RICE), see a doctor, and adjust workouts to meet recovery periods in the event of injuries.

People can create and carry out home exercise regimens that are customized to their requirements by taking these particular factors into account. This will improve physical fitness, general health, and overall well-being.

CHAPTER 9
Sophisticated Methods And Alternative Equipment

It can be quite helpful to incorporate advanced techniques and look into different equipment options to increase the variety and efficacy of at-home workouts. Targeting different muscle groups and enhancing overall strength and endurance can be accomplished with advanced bodyweight exercises and their variations, which are accessible yet tough. Exercises like pistol squats, one-arm push-ups, and plyometric jumps are fantastic additions to a home training regimen since they require more coordination and stability and work various muscle fibers.

By offering variable resistance and instability, respectively, the addition of stability balls and resistance bands to at-home workouts gives them a new dimension. Exercises like squats, rows, and chest presses can be made more difficult with resistance bands, providing a challenge that can be scaled to meet varying fitness levels.

However, stability balls work the core muscles, enhance posture, and increase balance, which makes exercises like planks, crunches, and bridges more interesting and dynamic.

A cheap and inventive method to increase the variety of workouts you can do at home is to repurpose everyday objects into fitness equipment. Exercises like weighted lunges, tricep dips, and bicep curls can be performed with objects like chairs, water bottles, and backpacks that hold books. This method not only reduces the cost of specialized equipment but also promotes creativity and ingenuity in creating training plans that are customized to each person's requirements and tastes.

Examining apps and virtual fitness courses is a practical and engaging method to get expert advice and inspiration while exercising at home. A variety of exercise programs are available on websites like YouTube, fitness applications, and online fitness forums. These include Pilates, yoga, high-intensity interval training (HIIT), and dance routines. Virtual courses frequently include qualified instructors, planned exercises, and immediate feedback, fostering a motivating atmosphere for reaching fitness objectives and maintaining consistency in at-home workouts.

Through the integration of sophisticated methods, investigation of alternative fitness equipment, inventive use of everyday objects, and participation in online fitness courses, people can optimize the efficiency and appeal of their at-home exercise regimens. These methods not only offer variation and challenge, but they also encourage regular exercise attendance, which enhances physical fitness, mental health, and general health.

CHAPTER 10
Long-Term Success And Sustainability

When starting a home exercise regimen, long-term success and sustainability become critical factors.

Sustainability is the capacity to continue working out regularly over an extended period, whereas long-term success involves reaching and maintaining fitness objectives that go beyond temporary benefits. These ideas are related since long-term success with at-home workouts frequently depends on sustainability.

Creating Long-Term Workout Routines at Home:

Developing a regimen that is pleasant, realistic, and flexible enough to change with the times is key to developing long-lasting at-home fitness habits. Setting attainable goals that meet your lifestyle limits and personal fitness aspirations is the first step.

Workout variation not only keeps things interesting but also pushes various muscle groups, improving overall fitness and avoiding plateaus.

The foundation of durable habits is consistency. Creating and adhering to a regular plan facilitates the integration of an exercise regimen into everyday life. Although it takes dedication and discipline, there are substantial benefits to both physical and mental health. Sustainability is further improved by including physical exercise into everyday habits, such as taking active breaks during sedentary times.

Including Days for Rest and Recovery:

Maintaining consistency is important, but so is giving the body enough time to rest and heal. Fatigue, a decline in performance, and an elevated risk of injury can result from overtraining. Rest days are crucial for refueling energy reserves, mending muscles, and preserving general health. Maintaining a balance between training volume and recovery days helps to sustain long-term results by reducing burnout and encouraging ongoing improvement.

On rest days, active rehabilitation techniques like gentle stretching or low-impact exercises might be helpful. It facilitates better circulation, lessens pain in the muscles, and speeds up recuperation without too stressing the body. Long-lasting fitness routines are facilitated by an awareness of personal recuperation requirements and the adaptation of training plans in response.

Seeking Assistance and Professional Guidance:

To maximize one's routines or for new individuals to at-home exercise, consulting a professional can be quite beneficial. Exercise physiologists and personal trainers are examples of fitness specialists who can offer encouragement, technical advice, and customized training schedules.

They also provide experience in creating progressive programs that guarantee ongoing advancement and avoid stagnation.

Including expert assistance could involve routine evaluations to monitor development, handle obstacles, and modify exercises as necessary. Additionally, by optimizing feeding techniques for performance and recuperation, nutrition advice from certified dietitians or nutritionists supports fitness activities.

Making use of internet resources, including reliable fitness websites or apps, can also offer helpful guidance and assistance.

Accepting a Lifetime of Health:

A lifetime commitment to exercise transcends passing trends and short-term objectives.

It requires embracing a way of thinking that sees physical exercise, well-being, and health as essential components of life. This change in perspective encourages a long-term approach to fitness, where working out becomes a habit as opposed to a chore.

A lifetime of fitness requires several essential elements, such as putting self-care first, having a positive outlook on exercise, and being flexible in the face of change. Flexible exercise programs can be modified to account for variations in age, fitness level, and lifestyle. Trying new sports or leisure pursuits is one way to add variety to your physical activity and avoid getting bored with your workouts.

Developing long-lasting routines, allowing time for relaxation and recuperation, obtaining expert advice, and accepting fitness as a lifelong adventure are all necessary for long-term success with at-home workouts. People can enjoy long-lasting improvements in their general quality of life, mental and physical health, and both by incorporating these ideas into their daily lives.

Summary

In-depth discussions of the complex relationship between mental health and physical fitness are covered in the book you're working on.

Subjects covered include the nature of mental health disorders and their effects, stress management techniques, coping mechanisms for anxiety and depression, the advantages of mindfulness and nutrition for mental health, the role that exercise plays in promoting mental health, the significance of sleep quality, resilience-building techniques, and real-life success stories that highlight the mind-body connection.